Smoothie Power Weight Loss Plan

I0436664

A Complete Action Plan for Losing Weight and Cleansing Your Body with Smoothies in 7 Days

By Emmanuel Joatham

Smoothie Power Weight Loss Plan

Smoothie Power Weight Loss Plan

By reading any document, the reader agrees that under no circumstances are we responsible for any losses, direct or indirect, which are incurred as a result of use of the information contained within this document, including – but not limited to errors, omissions, or inaccuracies.

Smoothie Power Weight Loss Plan

Recommended Products:

1. Sensational Smoothies - http://bit.ly/1rPjQjR
2. Reset 28 + 30-Day Whole Food Challenge Bundle - http://bit.ly/22dICXx
3. Smoothies Recipes: The Ultimate Guide to Making Delectable Smoothies at Home In Less Than 15 Minutes - http://amzn.to/1TVLCUX

For More Updates:

Visit my blog at: http://mysmoothiesecrets.com

Thank you for reading!

Table of Contents

Smoothie Power Weight Loss Plan

Introduction

Are you tired of trying diet after diet without getting any results? What if you could lose weight by drinking delicious homemade beverages? With a selection of tasty smoothie recipes, you can achieve your weight loss goals. Stop wasting your time and energy on fad diets. You are about to find out why smoothies offer a healthy alternative to traditional dieting options.

Discover the Cleansing Power of a Smoothie Detox

In the following pages, you will discover the power of cleansing with smoothies. By sticking to a list of carefully chosen smoothies, you can perform a healthy detox. This will get your digestive system moving and help promote weight loss.

Cardiovascular and Strength Training Exercises for Any Fitness Level

This guide will also provide you with easy to follow exercises that can increase your chances of success. Along with a healthy diet, you should incorporate moderate exercise into your routine.

Smoothie Power Weight Loss Plan

Learn How to Lose Weight with Delicious Smoothie Recipes

Anyone can get started on a smoothie diet, with the help of the Smoothie Weight Loss Action Plan. Step by step instructions will explain how to combine a smoothie detox, regular exercise, and smoothie replacement meals to reach your ideal weight as soon as possible. You will also find a great selection of 16 delicious smoothie recipes that you can easily whip together in just minutes.

Keep reading to learn how to lose weight with delicious smoothie recipes.

Smoothie Power Weight Loss Plan

<u>Chapter #1: The Power of Cleansing with Smoothies</u>

You have probably heard of detoxes and cleanses, without fully understanding how they work. A cleanse is not a cure-all solution to help you lose weight, but it can jump start your weight loss goals. Let us explore the actual power of cleansing with smoothies.

What is a Detox?

A detox, also known as a cleanse, is a way of ridding your body of harmful toxins and substances. When applied to food, a detox can help you to flush waste products. These detoxes generally last between 3 and 7 days, depending on your current health. During this period, you will eliminate solids from your diet, replacing your meals with healthy smoothies. When combined with proper hydration, you can cleanse your digestive system of waste that could be interfere with your weight loss goals.

Smoothie Power Weight Loss Plan

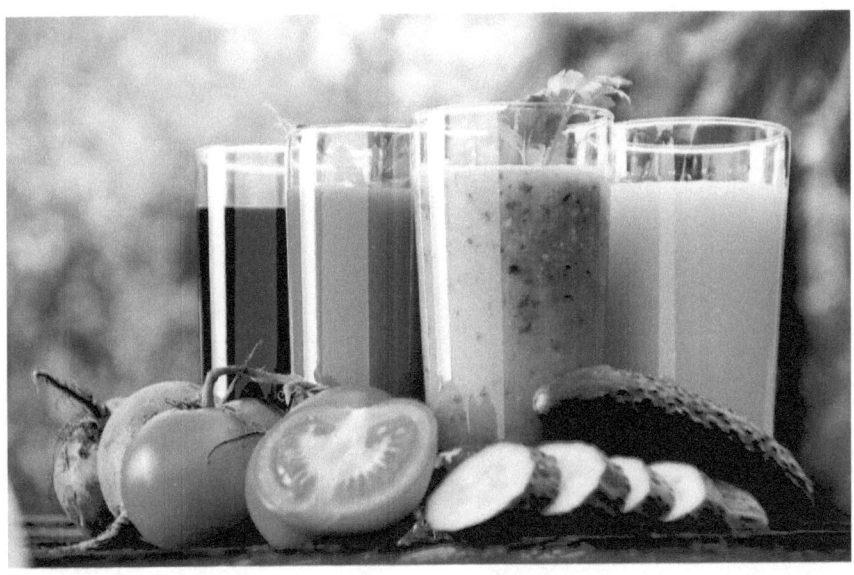

How Can a Detox Help You Lose Weight?

The main benefit of performing a detox is to give you a clean slate before starting a diet. Here is a breakdown of how this works:

- Speed up digestion by consuming liquid meals
- Eliminate unhealthy fats and unnecessary sugars
- Supply your body with proper hydration and nutrients
- Cleanse your liver and kidneys
- Improve your digestion and promote weight loss

Smoothie Power Weight Loss Plan

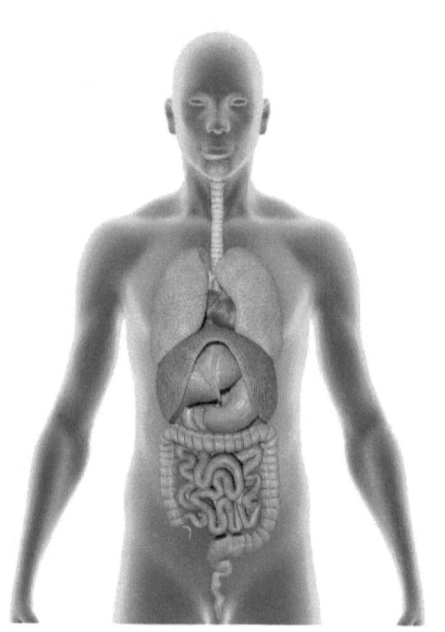

Essentially, you could perform a detox with any health foods and proper hydration. Though, receiving your nutrition in liquid form, such as from a smoothie, is easier on your digestive system.

When you consume solids, your digestive system has to break down the foods before the nutrients in the food can be absorbed. Once the food is broken down, waste is sent to your colon. Consuming a liquid meal speeds this process along, as your body does not have to break down the meal before sorting out the nutrients and the waste.

Also, by eliminating unhealthy fats and sugars, you are ensuring that your body receives optimal nutrition. There is less waste for your body to process when you eliminate processed foods and other unhealthy substances.

When performing a detox, it is important to stay hydrated. Drinking plenty of water helps the cleansing process. Many

Smoothie Power Weight Loss Plan

people notice a reduction in the frequency of headaches and fatigue when performing a detox. Another benefit that people often experience is regular bowel movements. These benefits are not actually the result of the detox, but the result of proper hydration.

After years of eating a diet full of processed foods, your liver and kidneys are working overtime. As harmful toxins and unhealthy substances build up in your kidneys and liver, these organs have more difficulty filtering waste. This can slow down your digestive process, making it more difficult to lose weight. A detox gives your kidneys and liver a break and cleanses them of these unhealthy substances.

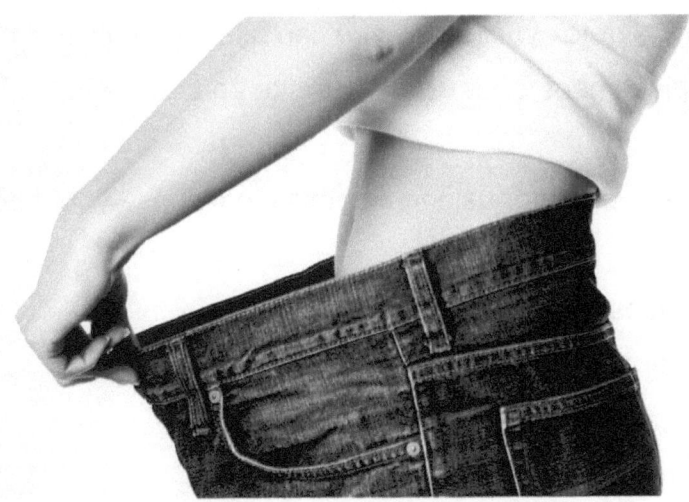

The combination of the effects described leads to improved digestion. The liquid smoothies are easier for your body to digest and allow your digestive process to flush out harmful toxins that could slow down your ability to lose weight.

The bottom line is that a detox gives you a good starting point for your diet. You should experience a substantial drop in weight after completing your detox. The average person loses between 2 and 5 pounds by performing a detox. Essentially, you can think of a detox as a reset for your digestive system.

Using Smoothies for a Detox

There are many different ways to cleanse your system, but a smoothie cleanse offers a healthy solution. Smoothies provide you with nutrition, as long as you select the right ingredients. If you want to detox your body, you can use smoothies as a meal replacement for several days – or up to a week.

There are 5 steps for using smoothies to cleanse your body:

1. Choose Your Smoothies
2. Prepare for the Detox
3. Drink 4 to 6 Smoothies Per Day
4. Drink Plenty of Water
5. Monitor Your Results

Smoothie Power Weight Loss Plan

Choose Your Smoothies

First, you will need to choose your smoothies. Towards the end of this guide, you will find a selection of healthy smoothie recipes. It is a good idea to include a large variety of smoothies in your diet while cleansing your system. You will be drinking between 4 and 6 smoothies per day.

If you are pressed for time, you could make 2 to 3 batches during the day, with each batch containing 2 servings. Just remember to store your second serving in an airtight container in your fridge. You may need to stir leftovers smoothies before serving.

Prepare for the Detox

About one week before starting your detox, you should prepare your body for the changes. Suddenly going from a diet full of processed foods to a diet containing only smoothies can be a shock to your system.

Prepare your body by replacing one meal per day with a smoothie. For example, one week before you start your detox, you could begin replacing your breakfast with a healthy smoothie from the selection of recipes provided later in this guide.

Smoothie Power Weight Loss Plan

Drink 4 to 6 Smoothies Per Day

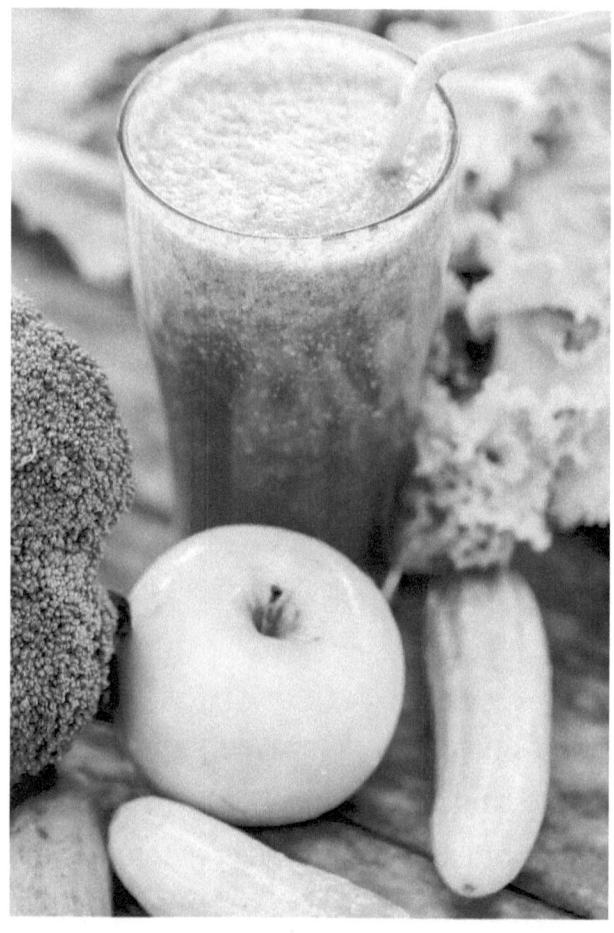

Once you are ready to get started on the cleanse, you will be drinking between 4 and 6 smoothies per day. It is important to include a variety of recipes so that your body receives proper nutrition. This also helps keep you from getting tired of drinking the same smoothies over and over again.

You should start your smoothie cleanse in the morning. Keep track of the day that you started and pay attention to your body. If you experience fatigue or weakness, you should return your normal diet. This is a rare occurrence and is often

Smoothie Power Weight Loss Plan

the result of eating a diet that primarily consists of starches and refined sugars.

Start your morning with a smoothie. The first smoothie of the day should include more fruit than vegetables. Fruit contains more sugar than vegetables, which gives your body energy for the day. Have another smoothie for lunch, 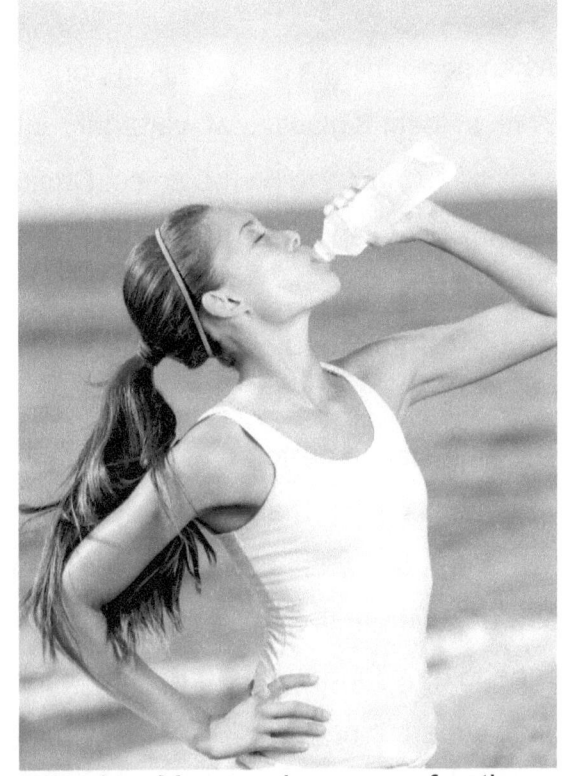 and another in the early evening. You can have your fourth smoothie when you would normally eat supper. You choose any of the smoothies provided later in this guide.

If 4 smoothies per day do not keep you full, then you can increase your daily smoothie count to 6. Several of these smoothies should contain blueberries, blackberries, or strawberries. Berries contain antioxidants which help promote the detoxification process.

http://mysmoothiesecrets.com © 2016

Smoothie Power Weight Loss Plan

Drink Plenty of Water

When performing a detox, it is important to stay hydrated. Drink at least 8 glasses of water throughout the day, in addition to your 4 to 6 smoothies. Drinking water will help you stay full between meals and also aid the cleansing process.

Monitor Your Results

The final step in performing a smoothie detox is to monitor your results. After the first couple of days, you should begin to notice some changes. You may experience more regular bowel movements and clearer urine. The length of detox will depend on your needs. Again, pay attention to your body. You should start to notice an increased energy, along with better focus and mental clarity. After several days, if you have not experienced any improvements or changes to your body, then you should continue with the detox. Continue drinking 4 to 6 smoothies per day for up to 7 days.

You may have trouble staying away from solids during your detox – especially during work. Snacking on some fresh fruit or vegetables during the day will not detract from your detox. You could snack on an orange, an apple, a banana, or any other fresh produce to keep you away from processed foods during the detox.

Smoothie Power Weight Loss Plan

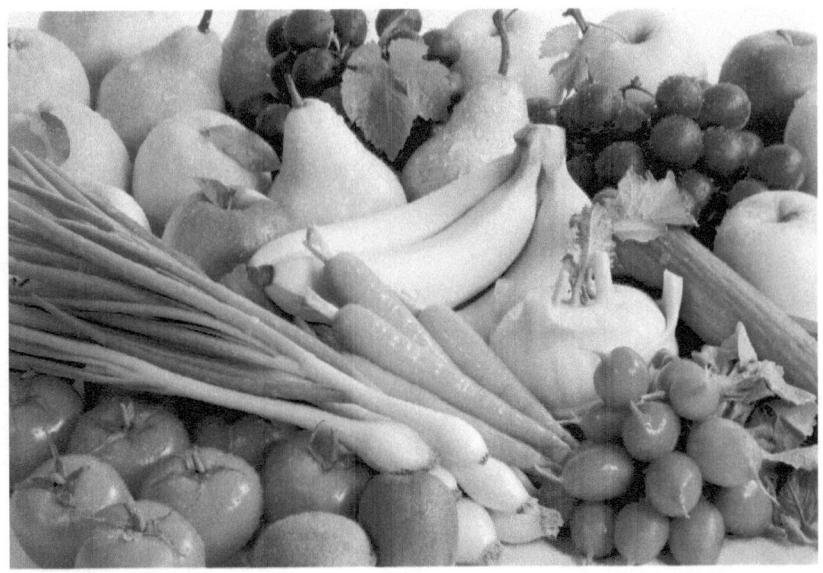

When the 3 to 7 days are up, you can resume your regular diet or use the Smoothie Weight Loss Action Plan provided later in this guide. If you are serious about weight loss, you should definitely consider using the easy-to-follow action plan.

Smoothie Power Weight Loss Plan

<u>Chapter #2: Exercises to Help Promote Weight Loss</u>

If you ask any doctor to describe the best method for losing weight they will likely tell you to eat a balanced diet and get regular exercise.

When you want to lose weight, you might focus solely on your diet. While eating healthy can help promote weight loss, you should make additional changes to your lifestyle and daily routine. Along with a healthy diet, you should include regular exercise.

You do not need to begin an intense workout to reach your ideal weight. But, it is a good idea to include some form of exercise. You can keep it simple. In the next chapter, you will create a 7-day workout schedule that you can use to promote weight loss, along with your smoothie diet.

So, which exercises should you use to lose weight? This will depend on your current fitness level and health. Workouts can be divided into two separate categories – cardiovascular exercises and strength training exercises.

Smoothie Power Weight Loss Plan

Cardiovascular Exercise

It is recommended that everyone gets 30 minutes of cardiovascular exercise at least 5 times per week. If you are not used to working out, this can seem like a lot of work. You can start off slowly. Choose a cardiovascular activity, such as:

- Walking
- Jogging
- Running
- Cycling
- Indoor cycling
- Swimming

For those that have not worked out in a while, you may want to start with walking. Whichever activity you choose you can start by performing 10 minutes of exercise Monday through Friday, for the first week. During your second week of exercise, increase your workout time to 20 minutes. When you reach the third week, switch to 30 minutes of exercise.

Smoothie Power Weight Loss Plan

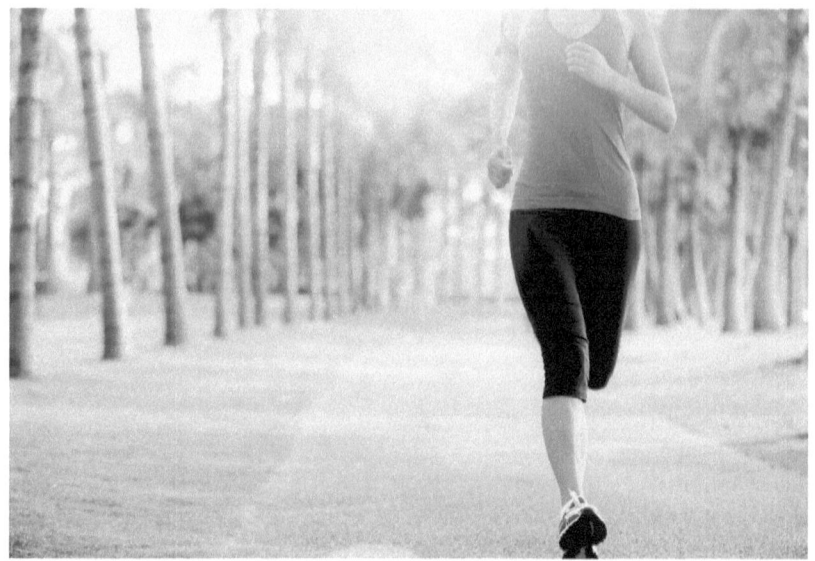

Cardiovascular exercise improves heart health and gets your blood pumping. You will burn additional calories, without engaging in a strenuous activity, and begin improving your overall health.

Strength Training Exercises

Cardiovascular exercise is a good place to start. If you really want to lose weight quickly and efficiently, then add strength training exercises to your routine. Again, you can start off slowly.

Smoothie Power Weight Loss Plan

Strength training helps you build muscle. While you do not need to develop large, bulging muscles, building some muscle definition will help you lose weight. The more muscle you have the more energy your body requires. Adding muscle increases your metabolism, allowing you to burn additional calories.

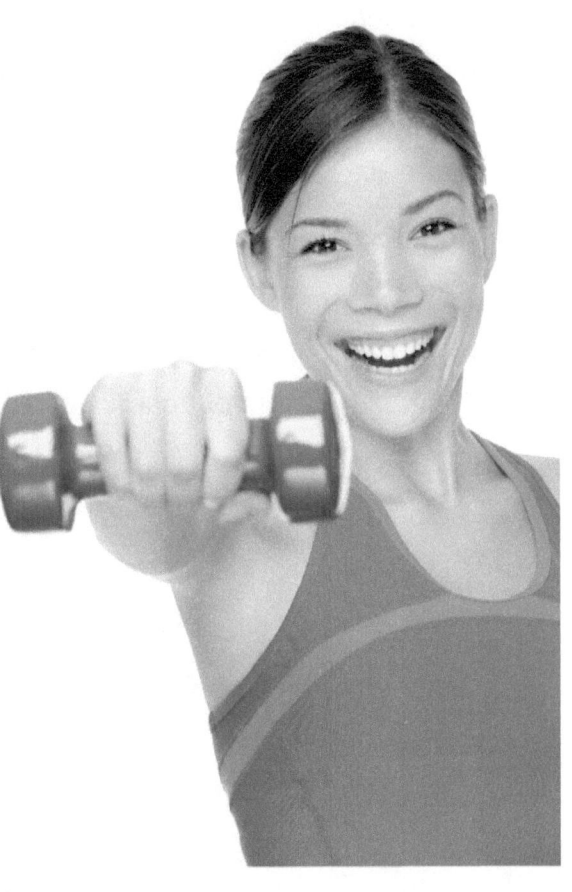

Perform a handful of strength training exercises after you complete your cardiovascular exercises for the day. By performing the cardio workouts first, you will improve blood circulation, which makes your strength training exercises more effective.

http://mysmoothiesecrets.com © 2016

Smoothie Power Weight Loss Plan

Spending 10 minutes performing strength training exercises will not take too much time out of your day. You could even shorten your cardio workout to 20 minutes so that your total workout only lasts 30 minutes.

5 Strength Training Exercises

Here are 5 strength training exercises that you can perform for about 10 minutes after your cardiovascular exercises:

- Dolphin Plank
- Single-Leg Dumbbell Row
- Squat to Overhead Press
- Step-Up with Bicep Curl
- Curtsy Lunge

Performing one set of each of the following exercises should take between 7 and 10 minutes. Depending on how long it takes to complete each exercise, you should include additional sets. Though, for the first few days, you should perform one set of each exercise to get a better sense of how long these strength training exercises take.

Smoothie Power Weight Loss Plan

Dolphin Plank

Lie face down on an exercise mat. Keep your toes tucked and your forearms on the floor next to your chest. Lift your belly button and raise your hips until you are in a plank position.

Inhale and lift your hips until your body forms the shape of an inverted V. Hold this pose for 1 second and then slowly return the starting plank position. Perform 15 repetitions to complete a set, which should take about 1 minute.

Single-Leg Dumbbell Row

The single-leg dumbbell row will work your shoulders, abs, biceps, quadriceps, and hamstrings. Stand up with a 5-pound weight in your left hand. Lean forward, with your right hand on a chair or structure for support. Continue leaning forward until your back is nearly parallel to the floor. As you lean forward, keep the weight in your left hand brought up towards your chest. After your back is mostly parallel, lower your left arm towards the floor. Lift your left leg behind you. Try to stretch your leg out in a straight line. This is the starting position.

Slowly bring your weight up, until your elbow is even with your torso. Hold for 1 second and then lower the weight. Perform

http://mysmoothiesecrets.com © 2016

15 repetitions and then switch sides for another 15 repetitions. One set should take about 2 minutes.

Squat to Overhead Press

For the squat to overhead press, you will stand with your feet shoulder-width apart. Your elbows should be bent with 5-pound weights in each hand at shoulder height. Your palms should be facing forward. Lower yourself into a squat and hold for 1 second.

Push through your heels to stand up. Press the weights over your head. Hold for 1 second and then return to the starting position. Perform 15 repetitions to complete a set. Each set should take a little over 1-minute.

Step-Up with Bicep Curl

The step-up with bicep curl will help work your hamstrings, biceps, quadriceps, and abs. Start with your left foot on a stool, bench, or chair. The surface should be stable and capable of supporting your entire weight. Hold a 5-pound weight in each hand.

In one motion, step your right foot onto the stool and then bring your right knee up until your thigh is parallel to the floor.

Smoothie Power Weight Loss Plan

As you perform this motion, you should lift the weights to perform a bicep curl. Step back down from the stool, with your left leg still on the chair. Perform 15 repetitions and then switch sides. One complete set, including both sides, should take about 2 minutes.

Curtsy Lunge

The final strength training exercise will help work your abs, along with your legs, hips, and butt. Stand with your feet hip-width apart. Your hands should be on your hips. Take a large step diagonally backward with your left foot and cross your left leg behind your right. As you step back, bend your knees and reach your left hand towards the floor, as you cross your left hand past the outside of your right foot. This motion is similar to performing a curtsy. Keep your right hand on your hip.

Return to the starting position and repeat for 15 repetitions before switching sides. Performing 15 repetitions on each side should take about 2 minutes.

Adding these 5 exercises to your schedule is not difficult. As mentioned, it should only take between 8 and 10 minutes to perform all of these exercises. After completing 20 to 30 minutes of cardio, you should perform at least 10 minutes of

http://mysmoothiesecrets.com © 2016

strength training. If you have the energy available, you could work out for longer.

Cut Back On Bad Habits

If you want to get the most out of your smoothie diet, you should incorporate additional healthy lifestyle choices. Cutting back on bad habits, such as smoking or drinking, getting enough rest, and staying hydrated can all help you reach your weight loss goals. Though, one of the greatest changes that you could make is to include regular exercise.

As you read through the Smoothie Weight Loss Action Plan provided in the next section, you will find out how to incorporate these exercises into your weight loss solution.

Combining exercise with a detox and healthy eating will help you get in the best shape of your life.

Smoothie Power Weight Loss Plan

Chapter #3: Smoothie Weight Loss Action Plan

Now that you understand the importance of regular exercise and performing a detox, it is time to explore the Smoothie Weight Loss Action Plan.

You will incorporate the tips provided in the previous chapters, along with a selection of tasty smoothie recipes found in the following chapter, to develop a plan for reaching your ideal weight. Everyone has different needs, goals, and personal preferences. For this reason, the Smoothie Weight Loss Action Plan has been made so that you can easily develop your own outline for losing weight with smoothies. The basis of this outline is a detailed weight loss journal.

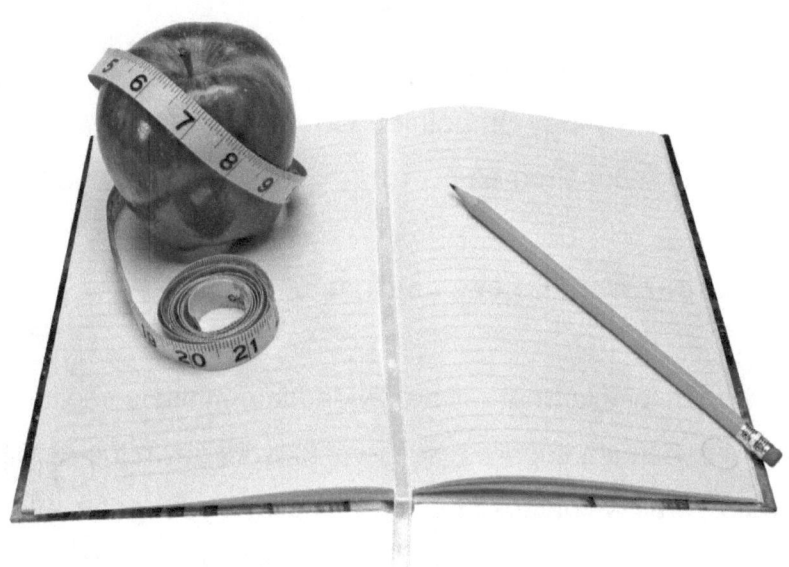

Smoothie Power Weight Loss Plan

Create a Weight Loss Journal

The first step to losing weight and getting in better shape is to create a weight loss journal. You can use a notebook or a word processing program on your computer. Your weight loss journal will include your goals, your workout schedule, and will provide a spot for you to log your progress.

Use the following steps to create a weight loss journal that includes a complete 7-day outline that you can follow week after week until you reach your ideal weight:

1. Outline Your Weight Loss Journal
2. Set Your Goals
3. Create a 7-Day Workout Schedule
4. Perform a 3 to 7-Day Cleanse
5. Create a 7-Day Smoothie Plan
6. Track Your Progress

Outline Your Weight Loss Journal

Your weight loss journal will be divided into multiple sections. You will use these separate sections to write down the details of your overall weight loss plan, starting with your goals and finishing with a section where you can track your progress. For each of the sections described below, start a new page in your

http://mysmoothiesecrets.com © 2016

journal, so that you have room to make adjustments and add in any notes.

Set Your Goals

Before you start detoxing your body or working out, you should set your goals. Decide on your ideal weight. You should also weigh yourself so that you have a starting figure to work with for tracking your progress. Weigh yourself in the morning, before you have had anything to eat. In addition to losing a specific amount of weight, you may have additional goals. This could include reaching a particular waist or dress size.

Write down your goals on the first page of your weight loss journal. This way, every time you open your journal, you are presented with your goals. It may also help to write down some of the reasons that you want to reach these goals, such as improved health, look better, feel healthier, prevent illness, or any other reasons that you may have for wanting to lose weight.

Create a 7-Day Workout Schedule

In order to create your 7-day workout schedule, refer back to the previous chapter and choose which exercise you would

Smoothie Power Weight Loss Plan

like to perform for your 20 minutes of cardiovascular exercise. Here are the options that you have to choose from:

- Walking
- Jogging
- Running
- Cycling
- Indoor cycling
- Swimming

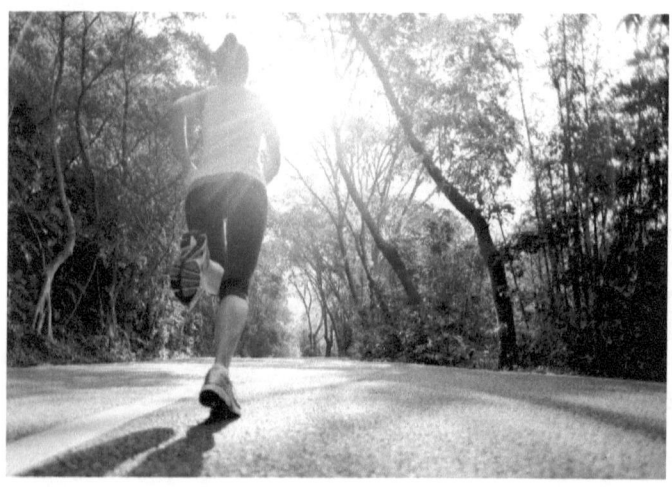 Choose one or more exercises that you would like to perform. If you have not worked out in a while, then you may want to start with walking. After several weeks, you could replace this with any of the other cardiovascular exercises. Along with choosing an exercise, you should choose two days of rest. Choose which 5 days of the week you want to exercise and which 2 days you want to rest. Write this down on a new page in your weight loss journal under a heading labeled "My Workout Schedule".

http://mysmoothiesecrets.com © 2016

Smoothie Power Weight Loss Plan

You will perform 20 minutes of cardiovascular exercise 5 days a week and rest for 2 days. In addition to cardiovascular exercise, you should include a selection of the strength training exercises described in the previous chapter. You should perform at least 10 minutes of strength training following your 20 minutes of cardiovascular exercise. Performing one set of each of the following exercises should take about 10 minutes. If you have the energy, you can add additional sets to your strength training workout – just pay attention to your body and avoid over-exerting yourself. Here are the strength training exercises that you should include in your workout:

- Dolphin Plank
- Single-Leg Dumbbell Row
- Squat to Overhead Press
- Step-Up with Bicep Curl
- Curtsy Lunge

Write down this list of exercises and the number of sets that you want to include in your workout. You can add this directly below your cardiovascular exercise in your weight loss journal.

Smoothie Power Weight Loss Plan

Perform a 3 to 7-Day Cleanse

Once you create a workout schedule, you can perform your smoothie cleanse. You should follow the instructions provided in the Power of Cleaning with Smoothies chapter.

Decide how long you want to perform the cleanse and write this down on a separate page in your weight loss journal. You should follow through with the detox for at least 3 days and up to 7 days. Again, remember to prepare your body for the detox. About one week before detoxing, you should begin replacing one of your meals with a smoothie.

Your detox will require you to drink between 4 and 6 smoothies per day. If you feel undernourished, you can include additional smoothies or snack on fresh fruits and vegetables during the day. Though, the fresh produce should be limited. The majority of your nutrition should come from the smoothies. The liquid smoothies are easier for your body to digest and process. This aids the cleansing process, so you will want to limit solid foods as much as possible.

Create a 7-Day Smoothie Plan

After completing the smoothie cleanse, you should get started on your smoothie diet. There really is not a whole lot to a

Smoothie Power Weight Loss Plan

smoothie diet. Basically, you will be replacing one or two meals per day with a smoothie while making better eating habits.

Here is a quick overview of the basic smoothie diet. You can make modifications to this based on your own individual needs:

1. Smoothie for Breakfast
2. Smoothie for Lunch
3. Healthy Protein Based Dinner
4. Light Snacks (Fruits, Vegetables, or Nuts) During the Day
5. Drink 8 Glasses of Water

Copy this information into your weight loss journal for easy reference. In the following chapter, you will find 16 delicious smoothie recipes. This provides you with enough variety to choose 2 separate smoothies for each day of the week, with 2 leftover recipes. You can follow the outline provided with the recipes or decide for yourself which smoothies you want to have for breakfast or lunch.

Smoothie Power Weight Loss Plan

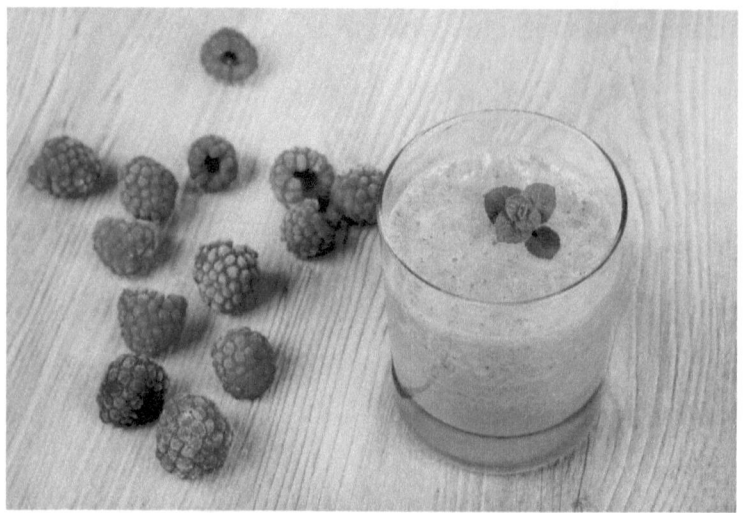

Have a smoothie for breakfast and a smoothie for lunch. These smoothies will give you all the energy you need to get through the day. You can use any of the smoothie recipes provided in the next chapter. Remember to include a variety of recipes in your diet, in order to provide you with optimal nutrition and keep you from getting bored of drinking the same smoothies every day. Again, you can follow the order that the recipes are listed or choose your own meal plan. If you decide to make your own meal plan based on the recipes provided, make sure that you write down the order in your weight loss journal.

For dinner, you should have a protein-based meal. This could include just about any meat dish, such as grilled chicken, salmon, or pork chops. Serve your meat with one to two servings of fresh or steamed vegetables. If you are a vegetarian, you should find healthy vegetarian meals that contain a good source of protein, such as meals made from tofu, lentils, or beans.

During the day, if you find yourself craving sugar or needing a snack, you can snack on fresh fruit, vegetables, seeds, or nuts. Pack one to two servings of one of these snacks and take it to work with you.

In addition to eating healthy, you should also drink healthy. Drink at least 8 glasses of water each day. Staying hydrated will also help promote digestive health and keep you full between meals.

Track Your Progress

The final part of the Smoothie Weight Loss Action Plan is to track your progress. Write down everything related to your weight loss activities in your journal. Write down what you eat each day, which exercises you perform, how long your workout lasts, and any extra details that you feel are relevant. The primary goal is to keep track of the steps that you are taking and to write down your results.

Smoothie Power Weight Loss Plan

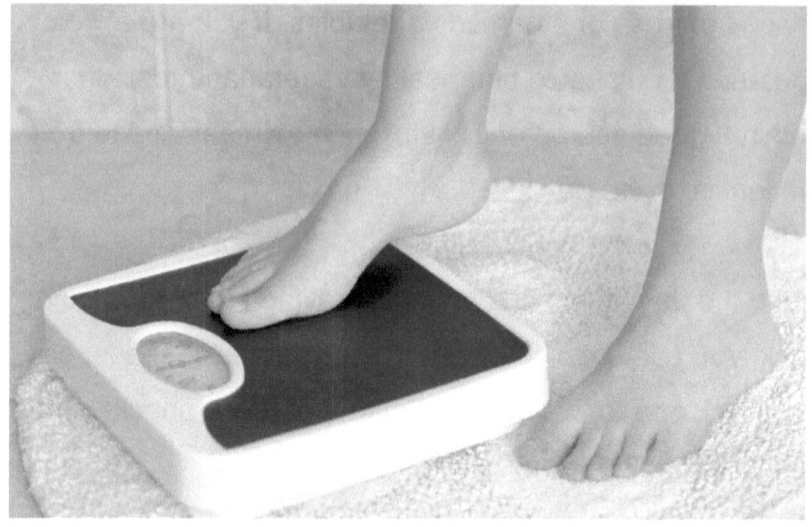

At the end of every week, you should perform a weigh-in. Do not weigh yourself more than once per week. The average person will lose between 1 and 2 pounds per week, with healthy eating and regular exercise. There will not be enough of a change day to day to be noticeable on the scales.

Write down the results of your weekly weigh-in and use this as motivation to keep up the good work. If you fall off the wagon, get right back up and continue with your plan the following day.

Smoothie Power Weight Loss Plan

<u>Chapter #4: Delicious Smoothie Recipes</u>

Smoothies are quick and easy to prepare, you just need to know which fresh fruits and vegetables to include. The following smoothie recipes can be used with the action plan provided in the previous chapter – or you can simply use these recipes for a tasty meal. In addition to the recipes listed below, you will also find tips and suggestions for making your own smoothie recipes.

Experiment with Different Combinations of Fruits and Vegetables

As you explore these various smoothie recipes, feel free to substitute any of the ingredients with a comparable fruit or vegetable. For example, if a recipe calls for kale, you could replace the kale with an equal amount of spinach. If the recipe calls for mango, you could replace with pineapple. Experiment with different combinations of fruits and vegetables.

You should also try new fruits and vegetables that you have not tried before. Every one to two weeks, when you go shopping for your produce, choose one fruit or vegetable that you have not tried before. Find a way to include this fruit or vegetable in the healthy recipes listed below or in a recipe of your own creation.

http://mysmoothiesecrets.com © 2016

Smoothie Power Weight Loss Plan

Now, on to the recipes. You will find 16 delicious smoothie recipes, all of which can be used as a part of the Smoothie Weight Loss Action Plan.

The instructions mostly the same for all of the recipes. You will first pour any liquids that are called for in the recipe into your blender. Then, add the fruit and vegetables. Some fruit and vegetables will need to be peeled or chopped prior to adding to your blender. For example, apples should be cored and peeled. After adding the liquid and produce, add any other ingredients that may be included, such as honey, ice, or various herbs and spices.

Blend until smooth and serve immediately. You can store leftovers in an airtight container, but you may need to stir the contents before serving. Some ingredients may require special preparation. For example, Chia seeds should be soaked overnight before using in a smoothie recipe.

Smoothie Power Weight Loss Plan

Day One Breakfast – Banana Oat Smoothie

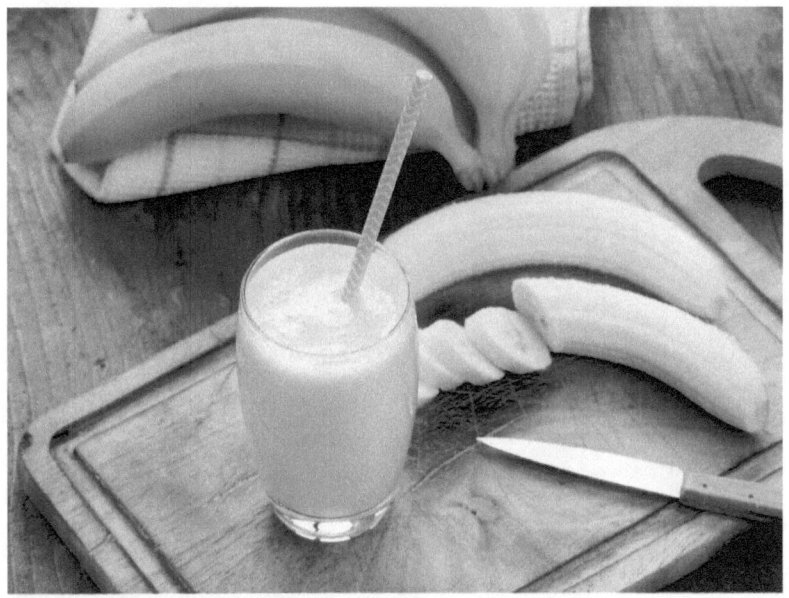

First up is the Banana Oat Smoothie. This recipe contains a good source of fiber and protein. The fiber from the oats and kefir will help get your digestive system moving. Here is the ingredients list – remember, simply combine the ingredients in your blender and blend until smooth:

- 1 banana
- ½ cup kale
- ¼ cup rolled oats
- 1 tablespoon Chia seeds (soaked overnight)
- 1 tablespoon almond butter
- ¼ teaspoon vanilla extract
- 1 pinch of cinnamon

http://mysmoothiesecrets.com © 2016

Smoothie Power Weight Loss Plan

Day One Lunch – Watermelon and Strawberry Smoothie

The Watermelon and Strawberry Smoothie is a refreshing drink. Have this for lunch or during the middle of the day. The sugar provided by the strawberries and melon will get you through the afternoon without causing a sugar crash. Here are 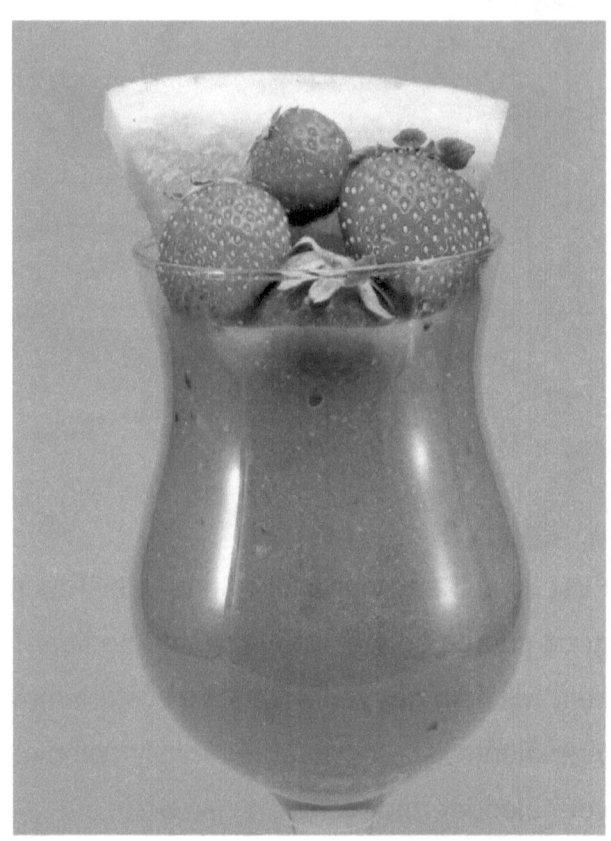 the ingredients needed for the Watermelon and Strawberry Smoothie:

- ¾ of a seedless watermelon
- ½ cup strawberries
- ½ cup spinach
- ½ cup plain yogurt
- 1/3 cup non-dairy milk

- 2 teaspoons vanilla extract
- 3 ice cubes

Day Two Breakfast – Peachy Morning Smoothie

The Peachy Morning Smoothie is another great option for starting your day. The inclusion of Chia seeds, which are to be soaked overnight, adds fiber to this smoothie. Use the following ingredients:

- 2 cups of spinach
- 1 peach
- 2 tablespoons Chia seeds
- ½ a frozen banana
- ½ an orange
- ¼ cup non-dairy milk (coconut, almond, or soy milk)

Day Two Lunch – Strawberry Banana Smoothie

This classic Strawberry Banana Smoothie is a perfect treat for any time of the day. Use it for a boost of energy before a workout or simply as a refreshing meal. Use the following ingredients to make your own Strawberry Banana Smoothie:

- ½ a frozen banana

Smoothie Power Weight Loss Plan

- ½ cup frozen strawberries
- ½ cup kale
- ½ cup kefir (or Greek yogurt)
- 1 tablespoon Chia seeds (soaked overnight)
- ½ cup almond milk
- 1 teaspoon vanilla extract

Day Three Breakfast – Orange Crush Smoothie

If you are in the mood for some orange, then try the Orange Crush Smoothie. This is a delicious smoothie with a creamy orange flavor. Here are the necessary ingredients:

- 1 orange
- 1 banana
- ½ cup spinach
- ½ cup non-dairy milk
- 1 teaspoon vanilla extract

Smoothie Power Weight Loss Plan

Day Three Lunch – Blueberry Lavender Smoothie

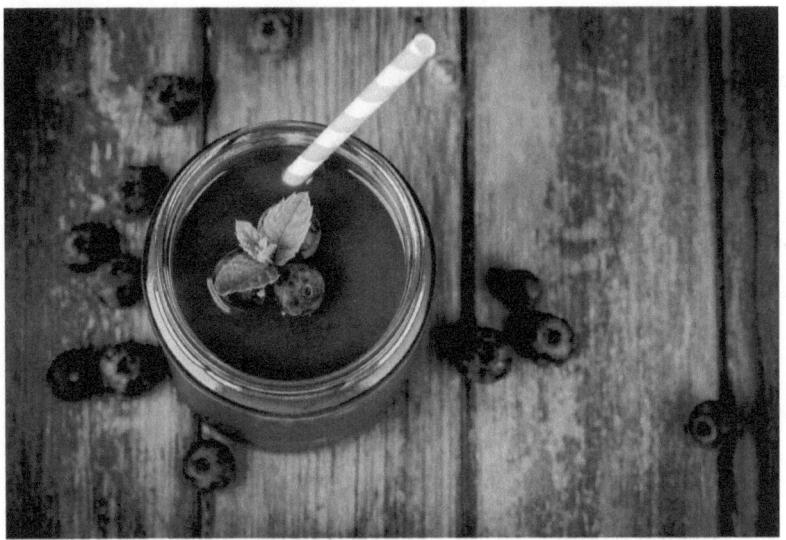

The Blueberry Lavender Smoothie can help increase your endurance. This makes the Blueberry Lavender Smoothie and ideal pre-workout drink. Use these ingredients:

- ½ cup frozen blueberries
- ½ a banana
- ½ cup almond milk
- ¼ cup water
- 1 teaspoon dried lavender
- 1 teaspoon vanilla extract

Smoothie Power Weight Loss Plan

Day Four Breakfast – Spicy Carrot Smoothie

The Spicy Carrot Smoothie includes cayenne pepper and ginger for an instant boost of energy. Cayenne pepper can help suppress your appetite and may be able to improve your metabolism. Here are the ingredients that you will need:

- 3 small carrots
- ½ cup avocado
- 1 tablespoon lemon juice
- ½ cup non-dairy milk
- 1 tablespoon freshly grated ginger
- 1 pinch of cayenne pepper

Day Four Lunch – Creamy Cantaloupe Smoothie

The Creamy Cantaloupe Smoothie is refreshing and light – perfect for a midday meal. Here are the ingredients needed for the Creamy Cantaloupe Smoothie:

- ½ a cantaloupe
- ½ cup Greek yogurt (plain)
- ½ cup spinach
- 1 tablespoon honey
- 3 ice cubes

http://mysmoothiesecrets.com © 2016

Smoothie Power Weight Loss Plan

Day Five Breakfast – Strawberry and Peach Smoothie

Enjoy a tasty Strawberry and Peach Smoothie any time of the day. Though, the nutrients will make a great start to your day. This smoothie will provide your body with an abundance of vitamin C and potassium. Here is the ingredient list:

- 1 cup frozen peach slices
- 1 cup fresh strawberries
- ½ cup Greek yogurt
- ½ teaspoon cinnamon
- 1 cup water (you can use non-dairy milk for a creamy smoothie)

http://mysmoothiesecrets.com © 2016

Smoothie Power Weight Loss Plan

Day Five Lunch – Cucumber and Spinach Smoothie

The Cucumber and Spinach Smoothie includes a variety of healthy green ingredients, along with some mango for added flavor. Use the following ingredients to prepare your Cucumber and Spinach Smoothie:

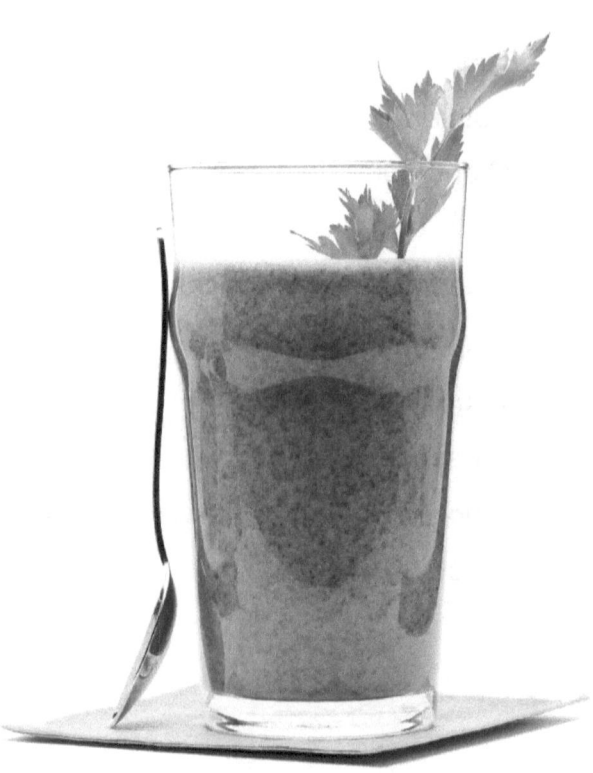

- 1 handful spinach
- 1/2 a mango (chopped)
- ½ cup coconut water (or coconut milk)
- 1 cup cucumber (chopped)
- ¼ jalapeno pepper (chopped)
- 1 small handful cilantro

http://mysmoothiesecrets.com © 2016

- 2 mint sprigs
- 1 lime (juiced)

Day Six Breakfast – Coconut Clementine Green Smoothie

This next smoothie also has a coconut flavor to it. This is an easy smoothie to prepare, but peeling the clementine may take a few minutes. Here is the ingredient list:

- 5 clementine (peeled)
- 1 banana
- ½ cup coconut milk
- 1 handful spinach
- 3 ice cubes

Smoothie Power Weight Loss Plan

Day Six Lunch – Ginger Pear Green Smoothie

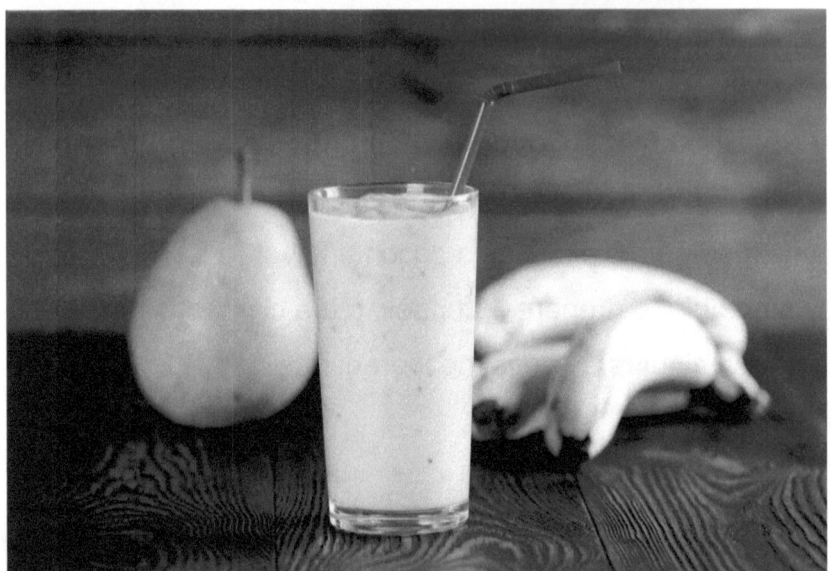

The Ginger Pear Green Smoothie will help with the detoxification process. Though, any of the smoothie recipes included in this guide can be used for your detox. Use the following ingredients:

- 1 large pear
- 1 ripe banana
- 2 handfuls of kale
- 1-inch of freshly grated ginger
- ½ cup coconut water

Smoothie Power Weight Loss Plan

Day Seven Breakfast – Mango Green Smoothie

The Mango Green Smoothie offers refreshment and a large dose of beneficial nutrients. This helps you start your day and gives you energy to get you through until lunch. Here are the ingredients that you will need:

- 1 ½ cups of frozen mango chunks
- 1 cup frozen strawberries
- 1 cup spinach
- 1 cup almond milk
- 1 frozen banana

Day Seven Lunch – Vanilla Lime Green Smoothie

The Vanilla Lime Green Smoothie has a tangy taste that is balanced with the inclusion of vanilla. The result is a creamy, decadent treat that is actually good for you. Use these ingredients to whip together your own Vanilla Lime Green Smoothie:

- ½ frozen banana
- ½ cup vanilla yogurt
- 1 cup spinach
- 2 tablespoons lime juice

http://mysmoothiesecrets.com © 2016

Smoothie Power Weight Loss Plan

- 2 teaspoons honey
- ½ teaspoon vanilla extract
- ½ cup non-dairy milk
- 4 ice cubes (optional)

Any Day – Spinach Orange Smoothie

The Spinach Orange Smoothie is a delicious drink that you can have any time of the day. It is a light meal, so it may be best for an afternoon snack. Here are the ingredients needed for the Spinach Orange Smoothie:

- 1 orange (peeled)
- ½ a frozen banana
- 1 cup spinach
- ¼ cup coconut water
- 1 tablespoon hemp or chia seeds (soaked overnight)
- 4 ice cubes

http://mysmoothiesecrets.com © 2016

Smoothie Power Weight Loss Plan

Any Day – Pina Colada Smoothie

The Pina Colada Smoothie provides a great way to end the day. After a long day of work, relax with the Pina Colada Smoothie. You will need the following ingredients:

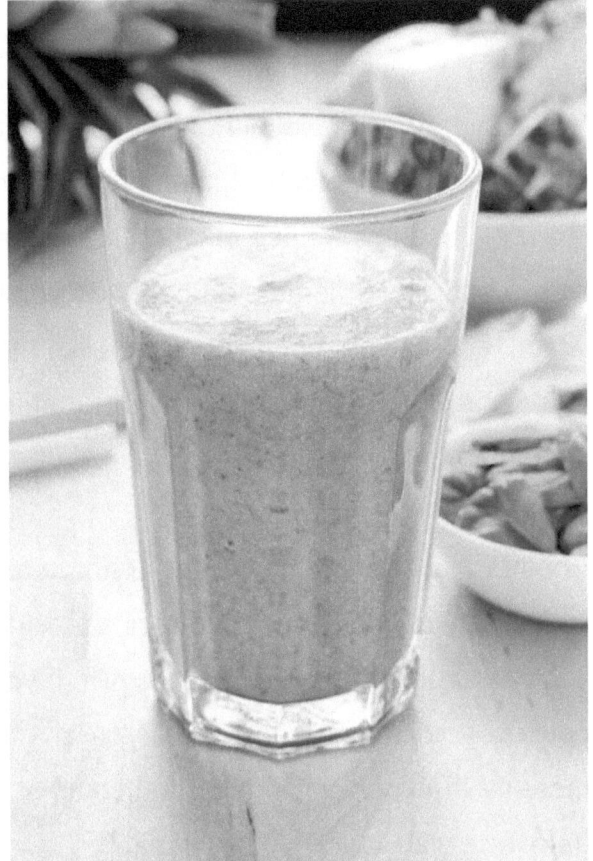

- ½ cup frozen pineapple
- ½ cup spinach
- 1 teaspoon honey
- 1 tablespoon shredded coconut
- ¼ teaspoon vanilla extract
- 1 cup coconut milk

http://mysmoothiesecrets.com © 2016

Smoothie Power Weight Loss Plan

Substituting Ingredients

You may have noticed by now that the majority of these recipes include spinach. Spinach and other green vegetables are often used as a base in smoothie recipes. They help create a thicker smoothie and provide you with essential vitamins and minerals. If you do not like the taste of spinach, you can replace with kale or any other nutritious green vegetable.

Another ingredient that you may want to substitute is non-dairy milk. Many of these smoothie recipes require non-dairy milk, such as coconut, almond, or soy milk. If you cannot find these options, you can use regular dairy milk. Though, dairy milk has more fat than non-dairy milk. You could also replace the non-dairy milk with water.

Smoothie Power Weight Loss Plan

Create Your Own Smoothie Recipes

Once you understand the basics of a standard smoothie recipe, it is relatively easy to make your 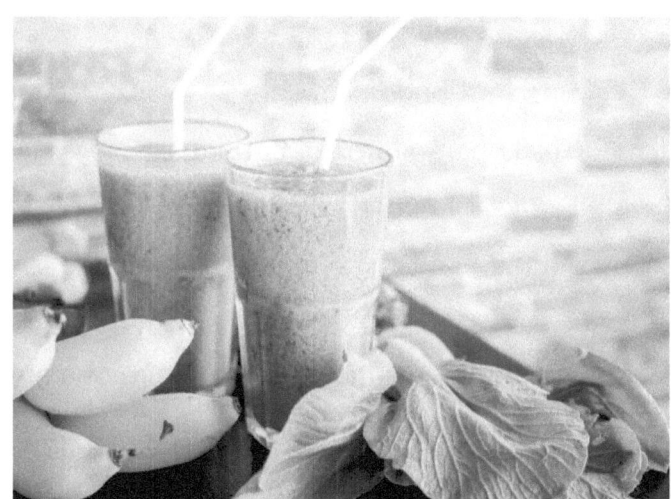 own. Here are the components of a typical smoothie:

- Base
- Thickener
- Liquid
- Added Flavoring

For the base, a vegetable is generally used, such as kale or spinach. The thickener is typically fresh or frozen fruit. Depending on the consistency of the fruit, liquid may also be needed to blend the ingredients together.

Non-dairy milk, such as soy, coconut, and almond milk are often used as the liquid ingredient. Added flavoring, such as a small amount of fruit, allows you to adjust the taste of the smoothie. Here is an example of an average smoothie recipe using these steps:

- Base – 1 handful of kale
- Thickener – 1 frozen banana
- Liquid – 1 cup of coconut milk
- Added Flavoring – ½ a fresh mango

Of course, this is just the basic structure of a smoothie recipe. You can add as many different ingredients as you would like, to create new and original smoothies.

Continue Trying New Smoothie Recipes

You should keep looking for new smoothie recipes and experiment with your own. A greater diversity will help keep your smoothie diet interesting and original.

Remember to incorporate these smoothie recipes into the Smoothie Weight Loss Action Plan. The recipes that have been chosen are all healthy, delicious smoothies that can help promote weight loss. The main goal, when selecting smoothies, is to choose recipes that are based around fruits and vegetables.

Smoothie Power Weight Loss Plan

As long as you do not add sugar, sweeteners, chocolate, whip cream, or other fattening fillers, then you should find that smoothies offer the best solution for losing weight. You can use smoothies for a detox, as outlined earlier, or use them to replace one or two meals during the day.

Enjoy these recipes, whether you choose to use the Smoothie Weight Loss Action Plan or simply want some tasty recipes.

Smoothie Power Weight Loss Plan
<u>Conclusion</u>

You now have the information needed to use smoothies as the ultimate weight loss tool. Smoothies offer the perfect solution for those that have struggled with weight loss. They are a great meal replacement.

The Ultimate Weight Loss Solution

By filling your body with healthy fruits and vegetables, you are supplying yourself with beneficial vitamins and minerals. When you include a variety of different smoothies in your diet, you are ensuring that you receive most of your nutrients. Smoothies are also easier for 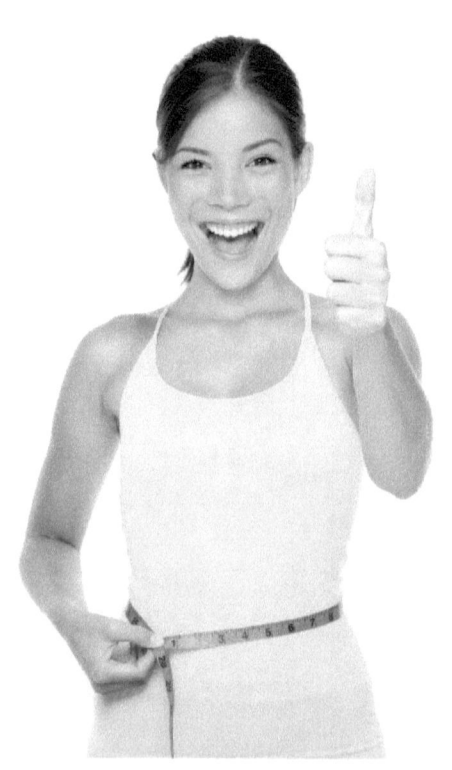 your body to digest than a solid meal. This makes smoothies great for cleansing your body, which will improve your

<u>http://mysmoothiesecrets.com</u> © 2016

digestion, boost your metabolism, and help you reach your weight loss goals.

Use the Smoothie Weight Loss Action Plan and the other suggestions in this guide to finally get in the best shape of your life. As you begin using the methods outlined in this guide, you may occasionally find it difficult to resist certain temptations, such as snacks or baked goods. If you stray from your smoothie diet, do not get discouraged. And, do not wait to get back on track.

Good luck on your smoothie diet! Have fun experimenting with different smoothie recipes and remember to try new fruits and vegetables.

Thank you for reading!